Special Chaffles Recipes

50 Special Chaffles Recipes for your Everyday Lifestyle

Imogene Cook

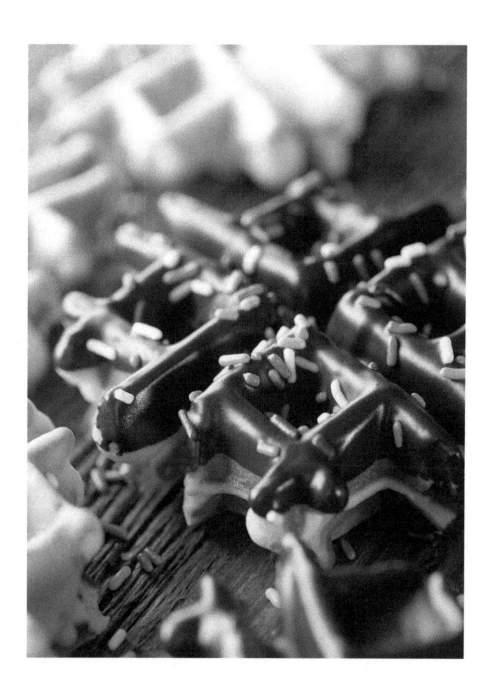

TABLE OF CONTENTS

How to Make Chaffles?

Equipment and Ingredients Discussed

Making chaffles requires five simple steps and nothing more than a waffle maker for flat chaffles and a waffle bowl maker for chaffle bowls.

To make chaffles, you will need two necessary ingredients –eggs and cheese. My preferred cheeses are cheddar cheese or mozzarella cheese. These melt quickly, making them the go-to for most recipes. Meanwhile, always ensure that your cheeses are finely grated or thinly sliced for use.

Now, to make a standard chaffle:

First, preheat your waffle maker until adequately hot.

Meanwhile, in a bowl, mix the egg with cheese on hand until well combined.

Open the iron, pour in a quarter or half of the mixture, and close.

Cook the chaffle for 5 to 7 minutes or until it is crispy.

Transfer the chaffle to a plate and allow cooling before serving.

11 Tips to Make Chaffles

My surefire ways to turn out the crispiest of chaffles:

Preheat Well: Yes! It sounds obvious to preheat the waffle iron before usage. However, preheating the iron moderately

will not get your chaffles as crispy as you will like. The best way to preheat before cooking is to ensure that the iron is very hot.

Not-So-Cheesy: Will you prefer to have your chaffles less cheesy? Then use mozzarella cheese.

Not-So Eggy: If you aren't comfortable with the smell of eggs in your chaffles, try using egg whites instead of egg yolks or whole eggs.

To Shred or to Slice: Many recipes call for shredded cheese when making chaffles, but I find sliced cheeses to offer crispier pieces. While I stick with mostly shredded cheese for convenience's sake, be at ease to use sliced cheese in the same quantity. When using sliced cheeses, arrange two to four pieces in the waffle iron, top with the beaten eggs, and some slices of the cheese. Cover and cook until crispy.

Shallower Irons: For better crisps on your chaffles, use shallower waffle irons as they cook easier and faster.

Layering: Don't fill up the waffle iron with too much batter. Work between a quarter and a half cup of total ingredients per batch for correctly done chaffles.

Patience: It is a virtue even when making chaffles. For the best results, allow the chaffles to sit in the iron for 5 to 7 minutes before serving.

No Peeking: 7 minutes isn't too much of a time to wait for the outcome of your chaffles, in my opinion.

Opening the iron and checking on the chaffle before

it is done stands you a worse chance of ruining it.

Crispy Cooling: For better crisp, I find that allowing the chaffles to cool further after they are transferred to a plate aids a lot.

Easy Cleaning: For the best cleanup, wet a paper towel and wipe the inner parts of the iron clean while still warm. Kindly note that the iron should be warm but not hot!

Brush It: Also, use a clean toothbrush to clean between the iron's teeth for a thorough cleanup. You may also use a dry, rough sponge to clean the iron while it is still warm.

Breakfast festive Chaffle Sandwich

Preparation time: 10 minutes

Cooking Time:10 Minutes

Servings: 2

Ingredients:

- 2 basics cooked chaffles
- Cooking spray
- 2 slices bacon
- 1 egg

Directions:

1. Spray your pan with oil.
2. Place it over medium heat.
3. Cook the bacon until golden and crispy.
4. Put the bacon on top of one chaffle.
5. In the same pan, cook the egg without mixing until the yolk is set.
6. Add the egg on top of the bacon.

7. Top with another chaffle.

Nutrition:

Calories 514 Total Fat 47 g Saturated Fat 27 g Cholesterol 274 mg Sodium 565 mg Potassium 106 mg Total Carbohydrate 2 g Dietary Fiber 1 g Protein 21 g Total Sugars 1 g

Cookie Dough Chaffle

Preparation time: 5 minutes

Cooking Time:7–9 Minutes

Servings: 2

Ingredients:

Batter

- 4 eggs
- ¼ cup heavy cream
- 1 teaspoon vanilla extract
- ¼ cup stevia
- 6 tablespoons coconut flour
- 1 teaspoon baking powder
- Pinch of salt
- ¼ cup unsweetened chocolate chips

Other

- 2 tablespoons cooking spray to brush the waffle maker
- ¼ cup heavy cream, whipped

Directions:

1. Preheat the waffle maker.
2. Add the eggs and heavy cream to a bowl and stir in the vanilla extract, stevia, coconut flour, baking powder, and salt. Mix until just combined.
3. Stir in the chocolate chips and combine.
4. Brush the heated waffle maker with cooking spray and add a few tablespoons of the batter.
5. Close the lid and cook for about 7–8 minutes depending on your waffle maker.
6. Serve with whipped cream on top.

Nutrition:

Calories 3, fat 32.3 g, carbs 12.6 g, sugar 0.5 g, Protein 9 g, sodium 117 mg

Thanksgiving Pumpkin Spice Chaffle

Preparation time: 5 minutes

Cooking Time:5minutes

Servings: 2

Ingredients:

- 1 cup egg whites
- ¼ cup pumpkin puree
- 2 tsps. pumpkin pie spice
- 2 tsps. coconut flour
- ½ tsp. vanilla
- 1 tsp. baking powder
- 1 tsp. baking soda
- 1/8 tsp cinnamon powder
- 1 cup mozzarella cheese, grated
- 1/2 tsp. garlic powder

Directions:

1. Switch on your square waffle maker. Spray with non-stick spray.
2. Beat egg whites with beater, until fluffy and white.
3. Add pumpkin puree, pumpkin pie spice, coconut flour in egg whites and beat again.
4. Stir in the cheese, cinnamon powder, garlic powder, baking soda, and powder.
5. Pour ½ of the batter in the waffle maker.
6. Close the maker and cook for about 3 minutes Utes.
7. Repeat with the remaining batter.
8. Remove chaffles from the maker.
9. Serve hot and enjoy!

Nutrition:

Protein: 51% 66 kcal Fat: 41% 53 kcal Carbohydrates: 8% kcal

Pumpkin Spice Chaffles

Preparation time: 10 minutes

Cooking Time: 14 Minutes

Servings: 2

Ingredients:

- 1 egg, beaten
- ½ tsp pumpkin pie spice
- ½ cup finely grated mozzarella cheese
- 1 tbsp sugar-free pumpkin puree

Directions:

1. Preheat the waffle iron.
2. In a medium bowl, mix all the ingredients.
3. Open the iron, pour in half of the batter, close, and cook until crispy, 6 to 7 minutes.
4. Remove the chaffle onto a plate and set aside.
5. Make another chaffle with the remaining batter.
6. Allow cooling and serve afterward.

Nutrition:

Calories 90 Fats 6.46g Carbs 1.98g Net Carbs 1.58g Protein 5.94g

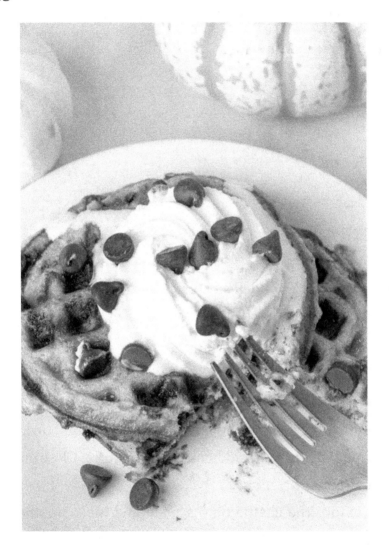

Chaffle Fruit Snacks

Preparation time: 10 minutes

Cooking Time: 14 Minutes

Servings: 2

Ingredients:

- 1 egg, beaten
- ½ cup finely grated cheddar cheese
- ½ cup Greek yogurt for topping
- 8 raspberries and blackberries for topping

Directions:

1. Preheat the waffle iron.
2. Mix the egg and cheddar cheese in a medium bowl.
3. Open the iron and add half of the mixture. Close and cook until crispy, 7 minutes.
4. Remove the chaffle onto a plate and make another with the remaining mixture.
5. Cut each chaffle into wedges and arrange on a plate.

6. Top each waffle with a tablespoon of yogurt and then two berries.

7. Serve afterward.

Nutrition:

Calories 207 Fats 15.29g Carbs 4.36g Net Carbs 3.g Protein 12.91g

Open-faced Ham & Green Bell Pepper Chaffle Sandwich

Preparation time: 10 minutes

Cooking Time: 10 Minutes

Servings: 2

Ingredients:

- 2 slices ham
- Cooking spray
- 1 green bell pepper, sliced into strips
- 2 slices cheese
- 1 tablespoon black olives, pitted and sliced
- 2 basic chaffles

Directions:

1. Cook the ham in a pan coated with oil over medium heat.
2. Next, cook the bell pepper.
3. Assemble the open-faced sandwich by topping each chaffle with ham and cheese, bell pepper and olives.

4. Toast in the oven until the cheese has melted a little.

Nutrition:

Calories 36 Total Fat 24.6g Saturated Fat 13.6g Cholesterol 91mg Sodium 1154mg Potassium 440mg Total Carbohydrate 8g Dietary Fiber 2.6g Protein 24.5g Total Sugars 6.3g

Taco Chaffle

Preparation time: 8 minutes

Cooking Time: 20 Minutes

Servings: 2

Ingredients:

- 1 tablespoon olive oil
- 1 lb. ground beef
- 1 teaspoon ground cumin
- 1 teaspoon chili powder
- ¼ teaspoon onion powder
- ½ teaspoon garlic powder
- Salt to taste
- 4 basic chaffles
- 1 cup cabbage, chopped
- 4 tablespoons salsa (sugar-free)

Directions:

1. Pour the olive oil into a pan over medium heat.
2. Add the ground beef.

3. Season with the salt and spices.Cook until brown and crumbly.
4. Fold the chaffle to create a "taco shell".
5. Stuff each chaffle taco with cabbage.
6. Top with the ground beef and salsa.

Nutrition:

Calories 255 Total Fat 10.9g Saturated Fat 3.2g Cholesterol 101mg Sodium 220mg Potassium 561mg Total Carbohydrate 3g Dietary Fiber 1g Protein 35.1g Total Sugars 1.3g

Choco Chaffle Cake

Servings:8

Cooking Time:5minutes

Ingredients:

- 8 keto chocolate square chaffles
- 2 cups peanut butter
- 16 oz. raspberries

Directions:

1. Assemble chaffles in layers.
2. Spread peanut butter in each layer.
3. Top with raspberries.
4. Enjoy cake on Christmas morning with keto coffee!

Nutrition:

Protein: 3% 1Kcal Fat: 94% 207 Kcal Carbohydrates: 3% 15 Kcal

Lt Chaffle Sandwich

Preparation time: 10 minutes

Cooking Time: 15 Minutes

Servings: 2

Ingredients:

- Cooking spray
- 4 slices bacon
- 1 tablespoon mayonnaise
- 4 basic chaffles
- 2 lettuce leaves
- 2 tomato slices

Directions:

1. Coat your pan with foil and place it over medium heat.
2. Cook the bacon until golden and crispy.
3. Spread mayo on top of the chaffle.
4. Top with the lettuce, bacon and tomato.
5. Top with another chaffle.

Nutrition:

Calories 238 Total Fat 18.4g Saturated Fat 5. Cholesterol 44mg Sodium 931mg Potassium 258mg Total Carbohydrate 3g Dietary Fiber 0.2g Protein 14.3g Total Sugars 0.9g

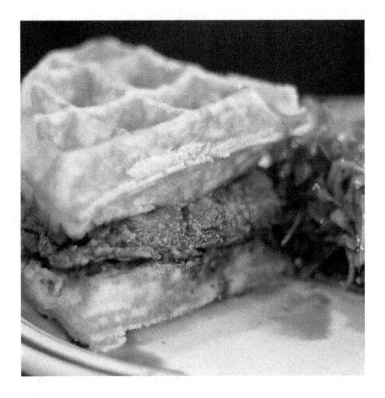

Mozzarella Peanut Butter Chaffle

Preparation time: 10 minutes

Cooking Time: 15 Minutes

Servings: 2

Ingredients:

- 1 egg, lightly beaten
- 2 tbsp peanut butter
- 2 tbsp Swerve
- 1/2 cup mozzarella cheese, shredded

Directions:

1. Preheat your waffle maker.
2. In a bowl, mix egg, cheese, Swerve, and peanut butter until well combined.
3. Spray waffle maker with cooking spray.
4. Pour half batter in the hot waffle maker and cook for minutes or until golden brown. Repeat with the remaining batter.
5. Serve and enjoy.

Nutrition:

Calories 150 Fat 11.5 carbohydrates 5.g Sugar 1.7 protein 8.8 cholesterol 86 mg

Double Decker Chaffle

Preparation time: 7 minutes

Cooking Time: 10 Minutes

Ingredients:

- 1 large egg
- 1 cup shredded cheese

TOPPING

- 1 keto chocolate ball
- 2 oz. cranberries
- 2 oz. blueberries
- 4 oz. cranberries puree

Directions:

1. Make 2 minutes dash waffles.
2. Put cranberries and blueberries in the freezer for about hours.
3. For serving, arrange keto chocolate ball between 2 chaffles.

4. Top with frozen berries,

5. Serve and enjoy!

Nutrition:

Protein: 23% 78 kcal Fat: % 223 kcal Carbohydrates: 9% 31 kcal

Cinnamon and Vanilla Chaffle

Preparation time: 5 minutes

Cooking Time:7–9 Minutes

Servings: 2

Ingredients:

Batter

- 4 eggs
- 4 ounces sour cream
- 1 teaspoon vanilla extract
- 1 teaspoon cinnamon
- ¼ cup stevia
- 5 tablespoons coconut flour

Other

- 2 tablespoons coconut oil to brush the waffle maker
- ½ teaspoon cinnamon for garnishing the chaffles

Directions:

1. Preheat the waffle maker.
2. Add the eggs and sour cream to a bowl and stir with a wire whisk until just combined.
3. Add the vanilla extract, cinnamon, and stevia and mix until combined.
4. Stir in the coconut flour and stir until combined.
5. Brush the heated waffle maker with coconut oil and add a few tablespoons of the batter.
6. Close the lid and cook for about 7–8 minutes depending on your waffle maker.
7. Serve and enjoy.

Nutrition:

Calories 224, fat 11 g, carbs 8.4 g, sugar 0.5 g, Protein 7.7 g, sodium 77 mg

New Year Cinnamon Chaffle With Coconut Cream

Preparation time: 7 minutes

Cooking Time: 5minutes

Servings: 2

Ingredients:

- 2 large eggs
- 1/8 cup almond flour
- 1 tsp. cinnamon powder
- 1 tsp. sea salt
- 1/2 tsp. baking soda
- 1 cup shredded mozzarella

FOR TOPPING

- 2 tbsps. coconut cream
- 1 tbsp. unsweetened chocolate sauce

Directions:

1. Preheat waffle maker according to the manufacturer's directions.
2. Mix together recipe ingredients in a mixing bowl.
3. Add cheese and mix well.
4. Pour about ½ cup mixture into the center of the waffle maker and cook for about 2-3 minutes Utes until golden and crispy.
5. Repeat with the remaining batter.
6. For serving, coat coconut cream over chaffles. Drizzle chocolate sauce over chaffle.
7. Freeze chaffle in the freezer for about10 minutes Utes.
8. Serve on Christmas morning and enjoy!

Nutrition:

Protein: 3 100 kcal Fat: 56% 145 kcal Carbohydrates: 5% 13 kcal

Chaffles And Ice-cream Platter

Preparation time: 10 minutes

Cooking Time:5 minutes

Servings: 2

Ingredients:

- 2 keto brownie chaffles
- 2 scoop vanilla keto ice cream
- 8 oz. strawberries, sliced
- keto chocolate sauce

Directions:

1. Arrange chaffles, ice-cream, strawberries slice in serving plate.
2. Drizzle chocolate sauce on top.
3. Serve and enjoy!

Nutrition: Protein: 26% kcal Fat: 68% 128 kcal Carbohydrates: 6% 11 kcal

Choco Chip Pumpkin Chaffle

Preparation time: 10 minutes

Cooking Time: 15 Minutes

Servings: 2

Ingredients:

- 1 egg, lightly beaten
- 1 tbsp almond flour
- 1 tbsp unsweetened chocolate chips
- 1/4 tsp pumpkin pie spice
- 2 tbsp Swerve
- 1 tbsp pumpkin puree
- 1/2 cup mozzarella cheese, shredded

Directions:

1. Preheat your waffle maker.
2. In a small bowl, mix egg and pumpkin puree.
3. Add pumpkin pie spice, Swerve, almond flour, and cheese and mix well.
4. Stir in chocolate chips.

5. Spray waffle maker with cooking spray.

6. Pour half batter in the hot waffle maker and cook for 4 minutes. Repeat with the remaining batter.

7. Serve and enjoy.

Nutrition:

Calories 130Fat 9.2 carbohydrates 5.9 sugar 0.6 protein 6.6 cholesterol mg

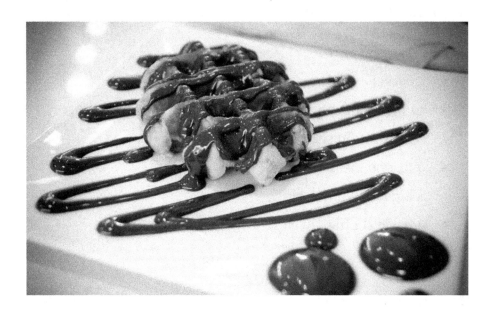

Sausage & Pepperoni Chaffle Sandwich

Preparation time: 8 minutes

Cooking Time: 10 Minutes

Servings: 2

Ingredients:

- Cooking spray
- 2 cervelat sausage, sliced into rounds
- 12 pieces pepperoni
- 6 mushroom slices
- 4 teaspoons mayonnaise
- 4 big white onion rings
- 4 basic chaffles

Directions:

1. Spray your skillet with oil.
2. Place over medium heat.
3. Cook the sausage until brown on both sides.
4. Transfer on a plate.

5. Cook the pepperoni and mushrooms for 2 minutes.
6. Spread mayo on top of the chaffle.
7. Top with the sausage, pepperoni, mushrooms and onion rings.
8. Top with another chaffle.

Nutrition:

Calories 373 Total Fat 24.4g Saturated Fat 6g Cholesterol 27mg Sodium 717mg Potassium 105mg Total Carbohydrate 28g Dietary Fiber 1.1g Protein 8.1g Total Sugars 4.5g

Pizza Flavored Chaffle

Preparation time: 6 minutes

Cooking Time: 12 Minutes

Servings: 2

Ingredients:

- 1 egg, beaten
- ½ cup cheddar cheese, shredded
- 2 tablespoons pepperoni, chopped
- 1 tablespoon keto marinara sauce
- 4 tablespoons almond flour
- 1 teaspoon baking powder
- ½ teaspoon dried Italian seasoning
- Parmesan cheese, grated

Directions:

1. Preheat your waffle maker.
2. In a bowl, mix the egg, cheddar cheese, pepperoni, marinara sauce, almond flour, baking powder and Italian seasoning.

3. Add the mixture to the waffle maker.

4. Close the device and cook for minutes.

5. Open it and transfer chaffle to a plate.

6. Let cool for 2 minutes.

7. Repeat the steps with the remaining batter.

8. Top with the grated Parmesan and serve.

Nutrition:

Calories 17 Total Fat 14.3g Saturated Fat 7.5g Cholesterol 118mg Sodium 300mg Potassium 326mg Total Carbohydrate 1.8g Dietary Fiber 0.1g Protein 11.1g Total Sugars 0.4g

Maple Chaffle

Preparation time: 10 minutes

Cooking Time: 15 Minutes

Servings: 2

Ingredients:

- 1 egg, lightly beaten
- 2 egg whites
- 1/2 tsp maple extract
- 2 tsp Swerve
- 1/2 tsp baking powder, gluten-free
- 2 tbsp almond milk
- 2 tbsp coconut flour

Directions:

1. Preheat your waffle maker.
2. In a bowl, whip egg whites until stiff peaks form.
3. Stir in maple extract, Swerve, baking powder, almond milk, coconut flour, and egg.
4. Spray waffle maker with cooking spray.

5. Pour half batter in the hot waffle maker and cook for 3-minutes or until golden brown. Repeat with the remaining batter.
6. Serve and enjoy.

Nutrition:

Calories 122 Fat 6.6 carbohydrates 9 sugar 1 protein 7 cholesterol 82 mg

Cinnamon Chaffle

Preparation time: 10 minutes

Cooking Time: 8 Minutes

Servings: 2

Ingredients:

- 1 egg
- ½ cup of mozzarella cheese, shredded
- 2 tablespoons almond flour
- 1 teaspoon baking powder
- 1 teaspoon vanilla
- 2 teaspoons cinnamon
- 1 teaspoon sweetener

Directions:

1. Preheat your waffle maker.
2. Beat the egg in a bowl.
3. Stir in the rest of the ingredients.
4. Transfer half of the batter into the waffle maker.
5. Close and cook for 4 minutes.

6. Open and put the waffle on a plate. Let cool for 2 minutes.
7. Do the same steps for the remaining batter.

Nutrition:

Calories 136 Total Fat 7.4g Saturated Fat 2.9g Cholesterol 171mg Sodium 152mg Potassium 590mg Total Carbohydrate 9.6g Dietary Fiber 3.6g Protein 9.9g Total Sugars 1g

Creamy Chaffles

Preparation time: 8 minutes

Cooking Time:5 minutes

Servings: 2

Ingredients:

- 1 cup egg whites
- 1 cup cheddar cheese, shredded
- 2 oz. cocoa powder.
- 1 pinch salt

TOPPING

- 4 oz. cream cheese
- Strawberries
- Blueberries
- Coconut flour

Directions:

1. Beat eggs whites with beater until fluffy and white
2. Chop Italian cheese with a knife and beat with egg whites.

3. Add cocoa powder and salt in mixture and again beat.

4. Spray round waffle maker non-stick cooking spray.

5. Pour batter in a round waffle maker.

6. Cook the chaffle for about 5 minutes Utes.

7. Once cooked carefully remove chaffle from the maker.

8. For serving, spread cream cheese on chaffle. Top with strawberries, blueberries and coconut flour.

9. Serve and enjoy!

Nutrition:

Protein: 26% 68 kcal Fat: 71% 187 kcal Carbohydrates: 3% 9 kcal

Choco And Spinach Chaffles

Preparation time: 10 minutes

Cooking Time:5 minutes

Servings: 2

Ingredients:

- 1 tbsp. almond flour
- ½ cup chopped spinach
- 1/2 cup cheddar cheese
- 1 tbsp. cocoa powder
- ½ tsp baking powder
- 1 large egg.
- 2 tbsps. almond butter
- 1/2 tsp salt
- 1/2 tsp pepper

Directions:

1. Preheat waffle iron while you are mixing the ingredients.
2. Blend all ingredients in a blender until mixed.
3. Pour 1/8 cup cheese in a waffle maker and then pour the

mixture in the center of greased waffle.

4. Again, sprinkle cheese on the batter.

5. Close the waffle maker.

6. Cook chaffles for about 4-5 minutes Utes until cooked and crispy.

7. Once chaffles are cooked remove and enjoy.

Nutrition:

Protein: 26% 4kcal Fat: 68% 128 kcal Carbohydrates: 6% 11 kcal

Pumpkin Chaffles With Choco Chips

Preparation time: 6 minutes

Cooking Time: 12 Minutes

Servings: 2

Ingredients:

- 1 egg
- ½ cup shredded mozzarella cheese
- 4 teaspoons pureed pumpkin
- ¼ teaspoon pumpkin pie spice
- 2 tablespoons sweetener
- 1 tablespoon almond flour
- 4 teaspoons chocolate chips (sugar-free)

Directions:

1. Turn your waffle maker on.
2. In a bowl, beat the egg and stir in the pureed pumpkin.
3. Mix well.

4. Add the rest of the ingredients one by one.

5. Pour 1/3 of the mixture to your waffle maker.

6. Cook for 4 minutes.

7. Repeat the same steps with the remaining mixture.

Nutrition:

Calories 93 Total Fat 7 g Saturated Fat 3 g Cholesterol 69 mg Sodium 13mg Potassium 48 mg Total Carbohydrate 2 g Dietary Fiber 1 g Protein 7 g Total Sugars 1 g

Red Velvet Chaffle

Preparation time: 6 minutes

Cooking Time: 12 Minutes

Servings: 2

Ingredients:

- 1 egg
- ¼ cup mozzarella cheese, shredded
- 1 oz. cream cheese
- 4 tablespoons almond flour
- 1 teaspoon baking powder
- 2 teaspoons sweetener
- 1 teaspoon red velvet extract
- 2 tablespoons cocoa powder

Directions:

1. Combine all the ingredients in a bowl.
2. Plug in your waffle maker.
3. Pour some of the batter into the waffle maker.
4. Seal and cook for minutes.

5. Open and transfer to a plate.

6. Repeat the steps with the remaining batter.

Nutrition:

Calories 126 Total Fat 10.1g Saturated Fat 3.4g Cholesterol 66mg Sodium 68mg Potassium 290mg Total Carbohydrate 6.5g Dietary Fiber 2.8g Protein 5.9g Total Sugars 0.2g

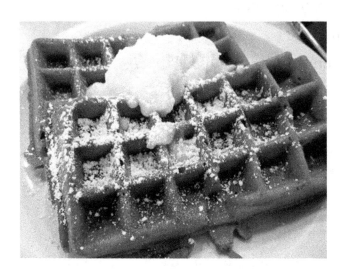

Walnuts Lowcarb Chaffles

Preparation time: 10 minutes

Cooking Time:5 minutes

Servings: 2

Ingredients:

- 2 tbsps. cream cheese
- ½ tsp almonds flour
- ¼ tsp. baking powder
- 1 large egg
- ¼ cup chopped walnuts
- Pinch of stevia extract powder

Directions:

1. Preheat your waffle maker.
2. Spray waffle maker with cooking spray.
3. In a bowl, add cream cheese, almond flour, baking powder, egg, walnuts, and stevia.
4. Mix all ingredients,

5. Spoon walnut batter in the waffle maker and cook for about 2-3 minutes Utes.

6. Let chaffles cool at room temperature before serving.

Nutrition:

Protein: 12% 11 kcal Fat: 80% kcal Carbohydrates: 8% 8 kcal

Chaffle Cream Cake

Servings: 8

Cooking Time: 30 Minutes

Ingredients:

Chaffle

- 4 oz. cream cheese
- 4 eggs
- 1 tablespoon butter, melted
- 1 teaspoon vanilla extract
- ½ teaspoon cinnamon
- 1 tablespoon sweetener
- 4 tablespoons coconut flour
- 1 tablespoon almond flour
- 1 ½ teaspoons baking powder
- 1 tablespoon coconut flakes (sugar-free)
- 1 tablespoon walnuts, chopped

Frosting

- 2 oz. cream cheese
- 2 tablespoons butter

- 2 tablespoons sweetener
- ½ teaspoon vanilla

Directions:

1. Combine all the chaffle ingredients except coconut flakes and walnuts in a blender.
2. Blend until smooth.
3. Plug in your waffle maker.
4. Add some of the mixture to the waffle maker.
5. Cook for 3 minutes.
6. Repeat steps until the remaining batter is used.
7. While letting the chaffles cool, make the frosting by combining all the ingredients.
8. Use a mixer to combine and turn frosting into fluffy consistency.
9. Spread the frosting on top of the chaffles.

Nutrition:

Calories127 Total Fat 13.7g Saturated Fat 9 g Cholesterol .9mg Sodium 107.3mg Potassium 457 mg Total Carbohydrate 5.5g Dietary Fiber 1.3g Protein 5.3g Total Sugars 1.5g

Simple Peanut Butter Chaffle

Preparation time: 5 minutes

Cooking Time:7–9 Minutes

Servings: 2

Ingredients:

Batter

- 4 eggs
- 2 ounces cream cheese, softened
- ¼ cup creamy peanut butter
- 1 teaspoon vanilla extract
- 2 tablespoons stevia
- 5 tablespoons almond flour

Other

- 1 tablespoon coconut oil to brush the waffle maker

Directions:

1. Preheat the waffle maker.

2. Add the eggs, cream cheese, and peanut butter to a bowl and stir with a wire whisk until just combined.

3. Add the vanilla extract and stevia and mix until combined.

4. Stir in the almond flour and stir until combined.

5. Brush the heated waffle maker with coconut oil and add a few tablespoons of the batter.

6. Close the lid and cook for about 7–8 minutes depending on your waffle maker.

7. Serve and enjoy.

Nutrition:

Calories 291, fat 24.9 g, carbs 5.9 g, sugar 2 g, Protein 12.5 g, sodium 1 mg

Beginner Brownies Chaffle

Preparation time: 10 minutes

Cooking Time:5 minutes

Servings: 2

Ingredients:

- 1 cup cheddar cheese
- 1 tbsp. cocoa powder
- ½ tsp baking powder
- 1 large egg.
- ¼ cup melted keto chocolate chips for topping

Directions:

1. Preheat dash minutes waffle iron and grease it.
2. Blend all ingredients in a blender until mixed.
3. Pour 1 tsp. cheese in a waffle maker and then pour the mixture in the center of greased waffle.
4. Again, sprinkle cheese on the batter.
5. Close the waffle maker.

6. Cook chaffles for about 4-5 minutes Utes until cooked and crispy.
7. Once chaffles are cooked remove.
8. Top with melted chocolate and enjoy!

Nutrition:

Protein: 24% 7kcal Fat: 72% 239 kcal Carbohydrates: 4% 14 kcal

Holidays Chaffles

Preparation time: 5 minutes

Cooking Time:5minutes

Servings: 2

Ingredients:

- 1 cup egg whites
- 2 tsps. coconut flour
- ½ tsp. Vanilla
- 1 tsp. baking powder
- 1 tsp. baking soda
- 1/8 tsp cinnamon powder
- 1 cup mozzarella cheese, grated

TOPPING

- Cranberries
- keto Chocolate sauce

Directions:

1. Make 4 minutes chaffles from the chaffle ingredients.
2. Top with chocolate sauce and cranberries
3. Serve hot and enjoy!

Nutrition:

Protein: 38% 133 kcal Fat: 57% 201 kcal Carbohydrates: 5% 18 kcal

Cherry Chocolate Chaffle

Preparation time: 10 minutes

Cooking Time: 10 Minutes

Servings: 2

Ingredients:

- 1 egg, lightly beaten
- 1 tbsp unsweetened chocolate chips
- 2 tbsp sugar-free cherry pie filling
- 2 tbsp heavy whipping cream
- 1/2 cup mozzarella cheese, shredded
- 1/2 tsp baking powder, gluten-free
- 1 tbsp Swerve
- 1 tbsp unsweetened cocoa powder
- 1 tbsp almond flour

Directions:

1. Preheat the waffle maker.
2. In a bowl, whisk together egg, cheese, baking powder, Swerve, cocoa powder, and almond flour.

3. Spray waffle maker with cooking spray.

4. Pour batter in the hot waffle maker and cook until golden brown.

5. Top with cherry pie filling, heavy whipping cream, and chocolate chips and serve.

Nutrition:

Calories 2Fat 22 carbohydrates 8.5 sugar 0.5 protein 12.7 cholesterol 212 mg

Bacon, Egg & Avocado Chaffle Sandwich

Preparation time: 10 minutes

Cooking Time: 10 Minutes

Servings: 2

Ingredients:

- Cooking spray
- 4 slices bacon
- 2 eggs
- ½ avocado, mashed
- 4 basic chaffles
- 2 leaves lettuce

Directions:

1. Coat your skillet with cooking spray.
2. Cook the bacon until golden and crisp.
3. Transfer into a paper towel lined plate.
4. Crack the eggs into the same pan and cook until firm.

5. Flip and cook until the yolk are set.

6. Spread the avocado on the chaffle.

7. Top with lettuce, egg and bacon.

8. Top with another chaffle.

Nutrition:

Calories 372 Total Fat 30.1g Saturated Fat 8.6g Cholesterol 205mg Sodium 3mg Total Carbohydrate 5.4g Dietary Fiber 3.4g Total Sugars 0.6g Protein 20.6g Potassium 524mg

Sausage & Egg Chaffle Sandwich

Preparation time: 10 minutes

Cooking Time: 10 Minutes

Servings: 2

Ingredients:

- 2 basics cooked chaffles
- 1 tablespoon olive oil
- 1 sausage, sliced into rounds
- 1 egg

Directions:

1. Pour olive oil into your pan over medium heat.
2. Put it over medium heat.
3. Add the sausage and cook until brown on both sides.
4. Put the sausage rounds on top of one chaffle.
5. Cook the egg in the same pan without mixing.
6. Place on top of the sausage rounds.
7. Top with another chaffle.

Nutrition:

Calories 332 Total Fat 21.6g Saturated Fat 4.4g Cholesterol 139mg Potassium 16g Sodium 463mg Total Carbohydrate 24.9g Dietary Fiber 0g Protein 10g Total Sugars 0.2g

Banana Nut Muffin

Preparation time: 6 minutes -4

Cooking Time: 12 Minutes

Servings: 2

Ingredients:

- 1 egg
- 1 oz. cream cheese
- ¼ cup mozzarella cheese, shredded
- 1 teaspoon banana extract
- 2 tablespoons sweetener
- 1 teaspoon baking powder
- 4 tablespoons almond flour
- 2 tablespoons walnuts, chopped

Directions:

1. Combine all the ingredients in a bowl.
2. Turn on the waffle maker.
3. Add the batter to the waffle maker.
4. Seal and cook for minutes.

5. Open and transfer the waffle to a plate. Let cool for 2 minutes.

6. Do the same steps with the remaining mixture.

Nutrition:

Calories 169 Total Fat 14g Saturated Fat 4.6g Cholesterol 99mgSodium 98mg Potassium 343mg Total Carbohydrate 5.6g Dietary Fiber 2g Protein 5g Total Sugars 0.6g

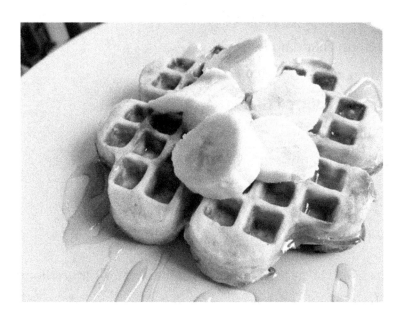

Cinnamon Roll Chaffles

Preparation time: 10 minutes

Cooking Time:5 minutes

Servings: 2

Ingredients:

- 1 tbsp. almond flour
- 1 tsp. cinnamon powder
- 1/2 cup cheddar cheese
- 1 tbsp. cocoa powder
- ½ tsp baking powder
- 1 large egg.
- 2 tbsps. peanut oil for topping

Directions:

1. Preheat waffle maker and mix together all ingredients in a bowl.
2. Pour the chaffle mixture in the center of the greased waffle maker.

3. Close the waffle maker.

4. Cook chaffles for about 5 minutes Utes until cooked and crispy.

5. Once chaffles are cooked, remove.

6. Pour melted butter oil on top.

7. Serve and enjoy!

Nutrition:

Protein: 15% 47 kcal Fat: % 247 kcal Carbohydrates: 3% 9 kcal

Choco Chip Lemon Chaffle

Preparation time: 10 minutes

Cooking Time: 15 Minutes

Servings: 2

Ingredients:

- 2 eggs, lightly beaten
- 1 tbsp unsweetened chocolate chips
- 2 tsp Swerve
- 1/2 tsp vanilla
- 1/2 tsp lemon extract
- 1/2 cup mozzarella cheese, shredded
- 2 tsp almond flour

Directions:

1. Preheat your waffle maker.
2. In a bowl, whisk eggs, Swerve, vanilla, lemon extract, cheese, and almond flour.
3. Add chocolate chips and stir well.
4. Spray waffle maker with cooking spray.

5. Pour 1/2 of the batter in the hot waffle maker and cook for 4-minutes or until golden brown. Repeat with the remaining batter.
6. Serve and enjoy.

Nutrition:

Calories 15at 10.8 carbohydrates 5.4 sugar 0.7 protein 9 cholesterol 167 mg

Crunchy Coconut Chaffles Cake

Preparation time: 5 minutes

Cooking Time: 15 Minutes

Servings: 2

Ingredients:

4 large eggs

1 cup shredded cheese

2 tbsps. coconut cream

2 tbsps. coconut flour.

1 tsp. stevia

TOPPING

1 cup heavy cream

8 oz. raspberries

4 oz. blueberries

2 oz. cherries

Directions:

1. Make 4 thin round chaffles with the chaffle ingredients. Once chaffles are cooked, set in layers on a plate.
2. Spread heavy cream in each layer.
3. Top with raspberries then blueberries and cherries.
4. Serve and enjoy!

Nutrition:

Protein: 21% 67 kcal Fat: 72% 230 kcal Carbohydrates: 7% 21 kcal

Coffee Flavored Chaffle

Preparation time: 5 minutes

Cooking Time: 7–9 Minutes

Servings: 2

Ingredients:

Batter

- 4 eggs
- 4 ounces cream cheese
- ½ teaspoon vanilla extract
- 6 tablespoons strong boiled espresso
- ¼ cup stevia
- ½ cup almond flour
- 1 teaspoon baking powder
- Pinch of salt

Other

- 2 tablespoons butter to brush the waffle maker

Directions:

1. Preheat the waffle maker.
2. Add the eggs and cream cheese to a bowl and stir in the vanilla extract, espresso, stevia, almond flour, baking powder and a pinch of salt.
3. Stir just until everything is combined and fully incorporated.
4. Brush the heated waffle maker with butter and add a few tablespoons of the batter.
5. Close the lid and cook for about 7–8 minutes depending on your waffle maker.
6. Serve and enjoy.

Nutrition:

Calories 300, fat 26.g, carbs 4.8 g, sugar 0.5 g, Protein 10.8 g, sodium 235 mg

Italian Sausage Chaffles

Preparation time: 10 minutes

Cooking Time: 8 Minutes

Servings: 2

Ingredients:

- 1 egg, beaten
- 1 cup cheddar cheese, shredded
- ¼ cup Parmesan cheese, grated
- 1 lb. Italian sausage, crumbled
- 2 teaspoons baking powder
- 1 cup almond flour

Directions:

1. Preheat your waffle maker.
2. Mix all the ingredients in a bowl.
3. Pour half of the mixture into the waffle maker.
4. Cover and cook for minutes.
5. Transfer to a plate.
6. Let cool to make it crispy.

7. Do the same steps to make the next chaffle?

Nutrition:

Calories 332 Total Fat 27.1g Saturated Fat 10.2g Cholesterol 9g Sodium 634mg Total Carbohydrate 1.9g Dietary Fiber 0.5g Total Sugars 0.1g Protein 19.6g Potassium 359mg

Chaffles With Strawberry Frosty

Preparation time: 7 minutes

Cooking Time: 5 Minutes

Servings: 2

Ingredients:

- 1 cup frozen strawberries
- 1/2 cup Heavy cream
- 1 tsp stevia
- 1 scoop protein powder
- 3 keto chaffles

Directions:

1. Mix together all ingredients in a mixing bowl.
2. Pour mixture in silicone molds and freeze in a freezer for about 4 hours to set.
3. Once frosty is set, top on keto chaffles and enjoy!

Nutrition:

Protein: 13% kcal Fat: 69% 99 kcal Carbohydrates: 18% 10 kcal

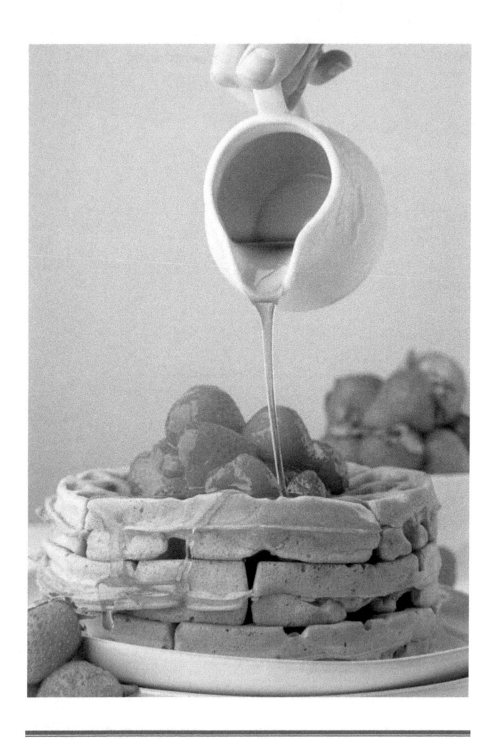

Pecan Pumpkin Chaffle

Preparation time: 10 minutes

Cooking Time: 15 Minutes

Servings: 2

Ingredients:

- 1 egg
- 2 tbsp pecans, toasted and chopped
- 2 tbsp almond flour
- 1 tsp erythritol
- 1/4 tsp pumpkin pie spice
- 1 tbsp pumpkin puree
- 1/2 cup mozzarella cheese, grated

Directions:

1. Preheat your waffle maker.
2. Beat egg in a small bowl.
3. Add remaining ingredients and mix well.
4. Spray waffle maker with cooking spray.

5. Pour half batter in the hot waffle maker and cook for minutes or until golden brown. Repeat with the remaining batter.
6. Serve and enjoy.

Nutrition:

Calories 121Fat 9.g Carbohydrates 5.7 sugar 3.3 protein 6.7 cholesterol 86 mg

Swiss Bacon Chaffle

Preparation time: 10 minutes

Cooking Time: 8 Minutes

Servings: 2

Ingredients:

- 1 egg
- ½ cup Swiss cheese
- 2 tablespoons cooked crumbled bacon

Directions:

1. Preheat your waffle maker.
2. Beat the egg in a bowl.
3. Stir in the cheese and bacon.
4. Pour half of the mixture into the device.
5. Close and cook for 4 minutes.
6. Cook the second chaffle using the same steps.

Nutrition:

Calories 23 Total Fat 17.6g Saturated Fat 8.1g Cholesterol 128mg Sodium 522mg Total Carbohydrate 1.9g Dietary Fiber 0g Total Sugars 0.5g Protein 17.1g Potassium 158mg

Bacon, Olives & Cheddar Chaffle

Preparation time: 10 minutes

Cooking Time: 8 Minutes

Servings: 2

Ingredients:

- 1 egg
- ½ cup cheddar cheese, shredded
- 1 tablespoon black olives, chopped
- 1 tablespoon bacon bits

Directions:

1. Plug in your waffle maker.
2. In a bowl, beat the egg and stir in the cheese.
3. Add the black olives and bacon bits.
4. Mix well.
5. Add half of the mixture into the waffle maker.
6. Cover and cook for 4 minutes.
7. Open and transfer to a plate.
8. Let cool for 2 minutes.
9. Cook the other chaffle using the remaining batter.

Nutrition:

Calories 202 Total Fat 16g Saturated Fat 8g Cholesterol 122mg Sodium 462mg Potassium 111mg Total Carbohydrate 0.9g Dietary Fiber 0.1g Protein 13.4g Total Sugars 0.3g

Garlic Chaffle

Preparation time: 10 minutes

Cooking Time: 8 Minutes

Servings: 2

Ingredients:

- 1 egg
- ½ cup cheddar cheese, beaten
- 1 teaspoon coconut flour
- Pinch garlic powder

Directions:

1. Plug in your waffle maker.
2. Beat the egg in a bowl.
3. Stir in the rest of the ingredients.
4. Pour half of the batter into your waffle maker.
5. Cook for 4 minutes.
6. Remove the waffle and let sit for 2 minutes.
7. Do the same steps with the remaining batter.

Nutrition:

Calories 170 Total Fat 14 g Saturated Fat 6 g Cholesterol 121 mg Sodium 220 mg Potassium 165 mg Total Carbohydrate 2 g Dietary Fiber 1 g Protein 10 g Total Sugars 1 g

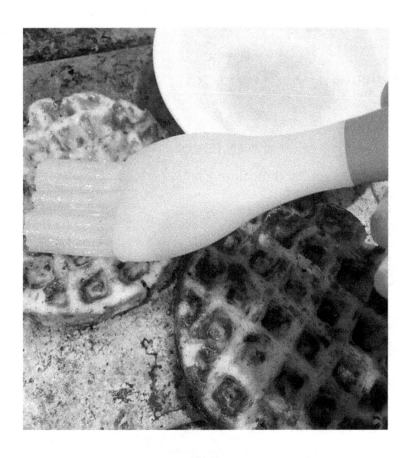

Herby Chaffle Snacks

Preparation time: 8 minutes

Cooking Time: 28 Minutes

Servings: 2

Ingredients:

- 1 egg, beaten
- ½ cup finely grated Monterey Jack cheese
- ¼ cup finely grated Parmesan cheese
- ½ tsp dried mixed herbs

Directions:

1. Preheat the waffle iron.
2. Mix all the ingredients in a medium bowl
3. Open the iron and pour in a quarter of the mixture. Close and cook until crispy, 7 minutes.
4. Remove the chaffle onto a plate and make 3 more with the rest of the ingredients.
5. Cut each chaffle into wedges and plate.
6. Allow cooling and serve.

Nutrition:

Calories 96Fats 6.29gCarbs 2.19gNet Carbs 2.19gProtein 42g

Zucchini Chaffle

Preparation time: 10 minutes

Cooking Time: 8 Minutes

Servings: 2

Ingredients:

- 1 cup zucchini, grated
- ¼ cup mozzarella cheese, shredded
- 1 egg, beaten
- ½ cup Parmesan cheese, shredded
- 1 teaspoon dried basil
- Salt and pepper to taste

Directions:

1. Preheat your waffle maker.
2. Sprinkle pinch of salt over the zucchini and mix.
3. Let sit for 2 minutes.
4. Wrap zucchini with paper towel and squeeze to get rid of water.
5. Transfer to a bowl and stir in the rest of the ingredients.

6. Pour half of the mixture into the waffle maker.

7. Close the device.

8. Cook for 4 minutes.

9. Make the second chaffle following the same steps.

Nutrition:

Calories 194 Total Fat 13 g Saturated Fat 7 g Cholesterol 115 mg Sodium 789 mg Potassium 223 mg Total Carbohydrate 4 g Dietary Fiber 1 g Protein 16 g Total Sugars 2 g

Breakfast Spinach Ricotta Chaffles

Preparation time: 8 minutes

Cooking Time: 28 Minutes

Servings: 2

Ingredients:

- 4 oz frozen spinach, thawed, squeezed dry
- 1 cup ricotta cheese
- 2 eggs, beaten
- ½ tsp garlic powder
- ¼ cup finely grated Pecorino Romano cheese
- ½ cup finely grated mozzarella cheese
- Salt and freshly ground black pepper to taste

Directions:

1. Preheat the waffle iron.
2. In a medium bowl, mix all the ingredients.
3. Open the iron, lightly grease with cooking spray and spoon in a quarter of the mixture.

4. Close the iron and cook until brown and crispy, 7 minutes.
5. Remove the chaffle onto a plate and set aside.
6. Make three more chaffles with the remaining mixture.
7. Allow cooling and serve afterward.

Nutrition:

Calories 1Fats 13.15gCarbs 5.06gNet Carbs 4.06gProtein 12.79g

Pumpkin Chaffle With Frosting

Preparation time: 10 minutes

Cooking Time: 15 Minutes

Servings: 2

Ingredients:

- 1 egg, lightly beaten
- 1 tbsp sugar-free pumpkin puree
- 1/4 tsp pumpkin pie spice
- 1/2 cup mozzarella cheese, shredded

For frosting:

- 1/2 tsp vanilla
- 2 tbsp Swerve
- 2 tbsp cream cheese, softened

Directions:

1. Preheat your waffle maker.
2. Add egg in a bowl and whisk well.
3. Add pumpkin puree, pumpkin pie spice, and cheese and stir well.

4. Spray waffle maker with cooking spray.

5. Pour 1/2 of the batter in the hot waffle maker and cook for 3-4 minutes or until golden brown. Repeat with the remaining batter.

6. In a small bowl, mix all frosting ingredients until smooth.

7. Add frosting on top of hot chaffles and serve.

Nutrition:

Calories 9at 7 carbohydrates 3.6 sugar 0.6 protein 5.6 cholesterol 97 mg

Chaffle Strawberry Sandwich

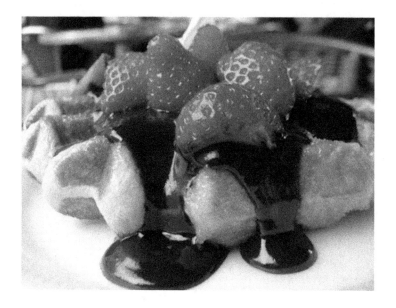

Preparation time: 7 minutes

Cooking Time: 5 Minutes

Servings: 2

Ingredients:

- 1/4 cup heavy cream
- 4 oz. strawberry slice

CHAFFLE Ingredients:

- 1 egg
- ½ cup mozzarella cheese

Directions:

1. Make 2 chaffles with chaffle ingredients
2. Meanwhile, mix together cream and strawberries.
3. Spread this mixture over chaffle slice.
4. Drizzle chocolate sauce over a sandwich.
5. Serve and enjoy!

Nutrition:

Protein: 18% 4kcal Fat: 78% 196 kcal Carbohydrates: 4% 10 kcal

Chocolate Chaffle

Preparation time: 10 minutes

Cooking Time: 8 Minutes

Ingredients:

- 1 egg
- ½ cup mozzarella cheese, shredded
- ½ teaspoon baking powder
- 2 tablespoons cocoa powder
- 2 tablespoons sweetener
- 2 tablespoons almond flour

Directions:

1. Turn your waffle maker on.
2. Beat the egg in a bowl.
3. Stir in the rest of the ingredients.
4. Put the mixture into the waffle maker.
5. Seal the device and cook for 4 minutes.
6. Open and transfer the chaffle to a plate to cool for 2 minutes.

7. Do the same steps using the remaining mixture.

Nutrition:

Calories 149 Total Fat 10. Saturated Fat 2.4g Cholesterol 86mg Sodium 80mg Potassium 291mg Total Carbohydrate 9g Dietary Fiber 4.1g Protein 8.8g Total Sugars 0.3g

New Year Keto Chaffle Cake

Servings:5

Cooking Time:15minutes

Ingredients:

- 4 oz. almond flour
- 2 cup cheddar cheese
- 5 eggs
- 1 tsp. stevia
- 2 tsp baking powder
- 2 tsp vanilla extract
- 1/4 cup almond butter, melted
- 3 tbsps. almond milk
- 1 cup cranberries
- I cup coconut cream

Directions:

1. Crack eggs in a small mixing bowl, mix the eggs, almond flour, stevia, and baking powder.
2. Add the melted butter slowly to the flour mixture, mix well to ensure a smooth consistency.

3. Add the cheese, almond milk, cranberries and vanilla to the flour and butter mixture be sure to mix well.

4. Preheat waffles maker according to manufacturer instruction and grease it with avocado oil.

5. Pour mixture into waffle maker and cook until golden brown.

6. Make 5 chaffles

7. Stag chaffles in a plate. Spread the cream all around.

8. Cut in slice and serve.

Nutrition:

Protein: 3% 15 Kcal Fat: % 207 Kcal Carbohydrates: 3% 15 Kcal

Thanksgiving Pumpkin Latte with Chaffles

Preparation time: 10 minutes

Cooking Time: 5 minutes

Servings: 2

Ingredients:

- 3/4 cup unsweetened coconut milk
- 2 tbsps. Heavy cream
- 2 tbsps. Pumpkin puree
- 1 tsp. stevia
- 1/4 tsp pumpkin spice
- 1/4 tsp Vanilla extract
- 1/4 cup espresso

FOR TOPPING

- 2 scoop whipped cream
- Pumpkin spice
- 2 heart shape minutes chaffles

Directions:

1. Mix together all recipe ingredients in mug and microwave for minutes Ute.
2. Pour the latte into a serving glass.
3. Top with a heavy cream scoop, pumpkin spice, and chaffle.
4. Serve and enjoy!

Nutrition:

Protein: 16 kcal Fat: 85% 259 kcal Carbohydrates: 10% 29 kcal

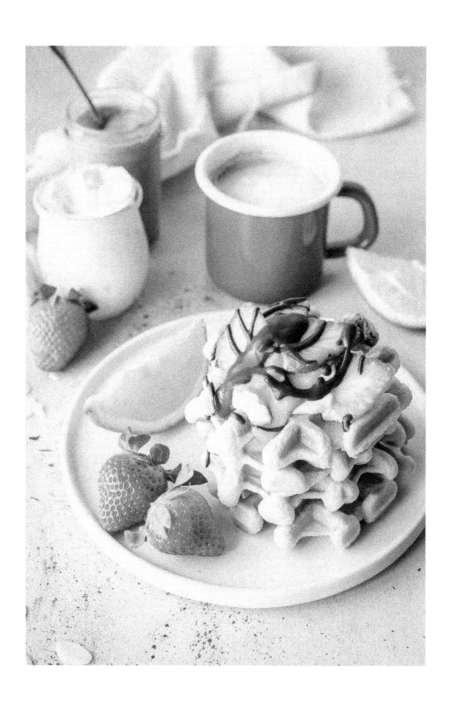

CPSIA information can be obtained
at www.ICGtesting.com
Printed in the USA
BVHW080812050521
606421BV00006B/1498

9 781802 771565